Health Tracker Belongs To

_____

_____

PERSONAL INFORMATION

NAME :

ADDRESS :

DATE OF BIRTH :

PLACE OF BIRTH :

MOBILE :   HOME :

EMAIL :

BLOOD GROUP :

WEIGHT :   HEIGHT :

EMERGENCY CONTACT

NAME :

ADDRESS :

MOBILE :   HOME :

EMAIL :

RELATIONSHIP :

NOTE

Contact person in last 7 days

_____

_____

_____

_____

_____

_____

_____

_____

_____

_____

_____

_____

_____

_____

_____

_____

_____

_____

_____

Place to visit in last 7 days

Important note

DAY 1

Date :

Symptoms

Note

DAY 2

Date :

Symptoms   :

_____

_____

_____

_____

_____

_____

_____

_____

_____

_____

_____

_____

_____

_____

_____

Note

_____

_____

_____

_____

_____

DAY 3

Date :

Symptoms

Note

DAY 4

Date :

Symptoms   :

Note

DAY 5

Date :

Symptoms

Note

DAY 6

Date :

Symptoms   :

Note

DAY 7

Date :

Symptoms

Note

DAY 8

Date :

Symptoms   :

Note

DAY 9

Date :

Symptoms

Note

DAY 10

Date :

Symptoms   :

Note

DAY 11

Date :

Symptoms

Note

DAY 12

Date :

Symptoms   :

Note

DAY 13

Date :

Symptoms

Note

DAY 14

Date :

Symptoms   :

Note

DAY 15

Date :

Symptoms

Note

DAY 16

Date :

Symptoms :

Note

DAY 17

Symptom Tracker

Date :

Symptoms

Note

DAY 18

Date :

Symptoms   :

Note

DAY 19

Symptom Tracker

Date :

Symptoms

Note

DAY 20

Date :

Symptoms   :

Note

DAY 21

Date :

Symptoms

Note

DAY 22

Date :

Symptoms   :

Note

Date :

Symptoms

_____

_____

_____

_____

_____

_____

_____

_____

_____

_____

_____

_____

_____

_____

Note

_____

_____

_____

_____

_____

DAY 24

Date :

Symptoms :

Note

DAY 25

Date :

Symptoms

Note

DAY 26

Date :

Symptoms :

Note

DAY 27

Date :

Symptoms

Note

DAY 28

Date :

Symptoms :

Note

DAY 29

Date :

Symptoms

Note

DAY 30

Date :

Symptoms   :

Note

DAY 1

Date :

Doctor / Hospital :

Medical Log

Note

DAY 2

Date :

Doctor / Hospital :

Medical Log

Note

DAY 3

Date :

Doctor / Hospital :

Medical Log

Note

DAY 4

Date :

Doctor / Hospital :

Medical Log

Note

DAY 5

Date :

Doctor / Hospital :

Medical Log

Note

DAY 6

Date :

Doctor / Hospital :

Medical Log

Note

DAY 7

Date :

Doctor / Hospital :

Medical Log

Note

DAY 8

Date :

Doctor / Hospital :

Medical Log

Note

DAY 9

Date :

Doctor / Hospital :

Medical Log

Note

DAY 10

Date :

Doctor / Hospital :

Medical Log

Note

DAY 11

Date :

Doctor / Hospital :

Medical Log

Note

DAY 12

Date :

Doctor / Hospital :

Medical Log

Note

DAY 13

Date :

Doctor / Hospital :

Medical Log

Note

DAY 14

Date :

Doctor / Hospital :

Medical Log

Note

DAY 15

Date :

Doctor / Hospital :

Medical Log

Note

DAY 16

Date :

Doctor / Hospital :

Medical Log

Note

DAY 17

Date :

Doctor / Hospital :

Medical Log

Note

DAY 18

Date :

Doctor / Hospital :

Medical Log

Note

DAY 19

Date :

Doctor / Hospital :

Medical Log

Note

DAY 20

Date :

Doctor / Hospital :

Medical Log

Note

DAY 21

Date :

Doctor / Hospital :

Medical Log

Note

DAY 22

Date :

Doctor / Hospital :

Medical Log

Note

DAY 23

Date :

Doctor / Hospital :

Medical Log

Note

DAY 24

Date :

Doctor / Hospital :

Medical Log

Note

DAY 25

Date :

Doctor / Hospital :

Medical Log

Note

DAY 26

Date :

Doctor / Hospital :

Medical Log

Note

DAY 27

Date :

Doctor / Hospital :

Medical Log

Note

DAY 28

Date :

Doctor / Hospital :

Medical Log

Note

DAY 29

Date :

Doctor / Hospital :

Medical Log

Note

DAY 30

Date :

Doctor / Hospital :

Medical Log

Note

Note

Note

Note

Note

Note

Made in the USA
Monee, IL
23 May 2020